YOUR KNOWLEDGE HAS VALUE

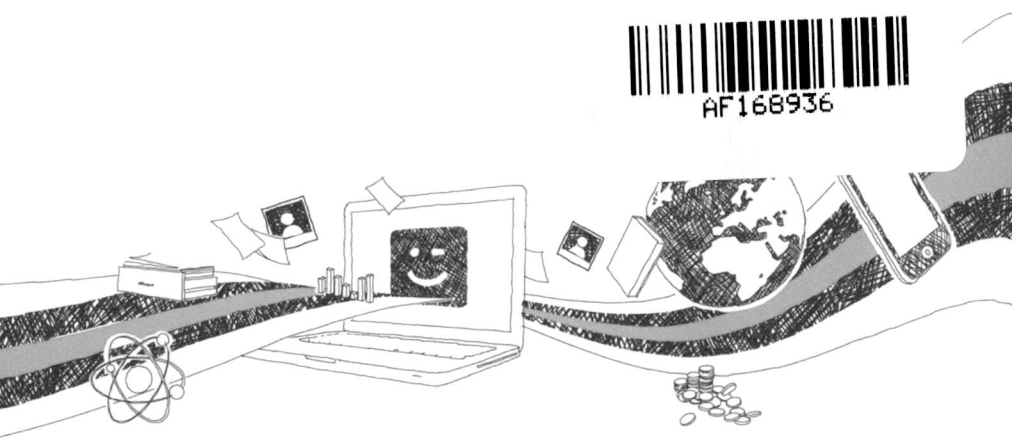

- We will publish your bachelor's and master's thesis, essays and papers

- Your own eBook and book - sold worldwide in all relevant shops

- Earn money with each sale

Upload your text at www.GRIN.com and publish for free

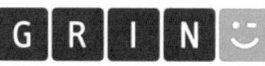

Bibliographic information published by the German National Library:

The German National Library lists this publication in the National Bibliography; detailed bibliographic data are available on the Internet at http://dnb.dnb.de .

This book is copyright material and must not be copied, reproduced, transferred, distributed, leased, licensed or publicly performed or used in any way except as specifically permitted in writing by the publishers, as allowed under the terms and conditions under which it was purchased or as strictly permitted by applicable copyright law. Any unauthorized distribution or use of this text may be a direct infringement of the author s and publisher s rights and those responsible may be liable in law accordingly.

Imprint:

Copyright © 2016 GRIN Verlag, Open Publishing GmbH
Print and binding: Books on Demand GmbH, Norderstedt Germany
ISBN: 9783668603899

This book at GRIN:

https://www.grin.com/document/381304

Patrick Kimuyu

Trauma Studies for Paramedics

GRIN Publishing

GRIN - Your knowledge has value

Since its foundation in 1998, GRIN has specialized in publishing academic texts by students, college teachers and other academics as e-book and printed book. The website www.grin.com is an ideal platform for presenting term papers, final papers, scientific essays, dissertations and specialist books.

Visit us on the internet:

http://www.grin.com/

http://www.facebook.com/grincom

http://www.twitter.com/grin_com

Trauma Studies for Paramedics

Name: Patrick K. Kimuyu

Question 1

Risks associated with treating a hypotensive patient with a penetrating chest wound inflicted by a 25cm blade using crystalloid fluids and alternative treatments available in pre-hospital setting

Fluids and venous therapy are still considered as essential elements of pre-hospital life support especially in critically ill patients. The initiation of fluid therapy should be based on clinical assessment in order to avoid the risk of hypovolaemic cardiac arrest during. Crystalloid fluids infusion offers a secure and safe brain through cerebral perfusion pressure. Secure brain function during injuries requires a systolic pressure of above 100mmHg (Søreide & Deakin, 2005). However, those patients' with severe brain injury are capable of tolerating low blood pressures. In the majority of pre-hospital setting, automated blood pressure gives erroneous values. The ideal pre-hospital fluid regime should combine hypertonic solution given during 10—20 minute's infusion and crystalloids or artificial colloids.

Researchers argue that the controversy surrounds the usage of crystalloid fluids in balancing tissue oxygen delivery against increasing the blood loss especially to patients with uncontrolled hemorrhage. These fluids are not capable of checking uncontrolled bleeding that occurs in multiple sites. As a result, patients' are exposed to severe bleeding capable of leading to hypovolaemic cardiac arrest This is trauma resulting from chest wound compromises tissue oxygenation resulting to hemorrhage (Søreide & Deakin, 2005). More importantly, blunt trauma lead to tissue edema, pain, neurogenic factors and spinal injury hence the likelihood of circulatory failure in such patients.

Intravenous fluids can cause haemodilution increment in the extra-cellular fluid compartment. Ideally, researchers argue that the relative expansion of the intravascular volume with 500 ml of an isotonic crystalloid is greater in shocked patients compared to healthy volunteers. Though is vital to raise the systolic pressure especially for the injured brain, there is a high risk of disruption of haemostatic clots in damaged blood vessels resulting to further bleeding (Søreide & Deakin, 2005).

It is also believed that the usage of crystalloid fluids leads to tissue edema, which has the potential of interfering with gaseous exchange in the lungs. Since the establishment of pre-hospital fluid therapy might delay transport and definite medical intervention, such patients are more likely to die before reaching hospitals. Research also indicates that crystalloid fluids increase bacterial translocation in the gut resulting to reduction in capillary blood flow. These effects are fatal given the conditions which prevail in many pre-hospital establishments. According to Søreide and Deakin (2005), the usage of crystalloid fluids in pre-hospital setting raises the possibility if suffering from renal impairment and allergy reaction hence the need to use them with absolute care.

Based on the uncertainties that surround the usage of crystalloid fluids in pre-hospital setting, it is recommended to adopt hypertonic saline. Hypertonic saline osmotic properties attract fluid in the intravascular compartment, and the addition of dextran helps in prolonging this effect by binding to recruited water. Such fluid has been found to improve hemodynamics and rapid adjustment of the blood pressure. Additionally, utilizing artificial oxygen carriers will help in keeping the cardiac output adequate (Søreide & Deakin, 2005). Basically, trauma impairs the oxygen-carrying capacity of the blood affecting brain functioning.

Question 2

Focused Assessment with Sonography in Trauma (F.A.S.T.) has been adopted in battlefield trauma care. Support or refute it application in civilian pre-hospital care.

According to Rose (2004), exsanguinations from injuries and organs of the abdomen, liver, spleen and kidney remains one of the reasons for high mortality after trauma. Blunt abdominal trauma is mostly caused by vehicle accidents, fall and blows involving the abdomen. The assessment of abdominal injury is a challenge to the medical fraternity owing to the presence of other injuries and alteration of mental status of the affected patients. FAST was adopted in the medical field in 1990's following the inefficiency of diagnostic peritoneal lavage. Initially, the technique was seen as non-invasive, accurate and offered expedient aid in decision-making processes in cases that required further treatment. In the modern world, FAST is widely used by physicians and surgeons in the emergency department (Rose, 2004).

FAST is also used in the primary circulatory survey to those patients' who have sustained blunt abdominal trauma so as to help in detecting pericardial and intraperitoneal fluids. FAST is also used in assessing the thoracic cavity for pneumothorax. Rose (2004) believes that FAST is easy to use, easily available and has low-cost imaging hence making the technique popular in the medical setting. The procedure offers greater flexibility that enables patients' to change positions, and this is critical for those patients who have undergone significant trauma. The procedure can be carried out simultaneously with diagnostic and therapeutic tests

According to Rose (2004), those patients' with positive FAST results have a high mortality rate compared to FAST negative patients'. As a result, FAST is an effective method in identifying those patients with the risk of serious intra-abdominal injuries. Additionally, FAST results can be used in guiding mobilization of the hospital resources and identify those patients' who can be managed expectantly. However, despite the beneficial aspect of FAST, researchers hold that the technique does not detect the exact site of organ injury. This implies that positive FAST patient is supposed to go for CT scans in order to locate the site of bleeding and extend of injury. Additionally, the sensitivity nature of FAST is low compared to other imaging modalities. Other limitations such as the inability to standardize the procedure, poor scanning results, especially in patients' with tissue abnormalities affects the reliability of the results (Rose, 2004)..

Due to various question regarding the next action following negative FAST results for hemoperitoneum, the procedure is slowly losing its usage in civilian pre-hospital settings. Many people have turned to CT scanning since it is widely available, fast and economical in such situations. CT scans dominate in many abdominal trauma patients. The technique is more accurate than FAST especially when comparing false negative rates of tests. Rose (2004) observes that the discordance in FAST result has forced many centers to adopt CT scans as their primary modality for their blunt abdominal trauma. Research also indicate that a clinical suspicion remain in determining therapeutic steps in trauma patients. For instance, a negative seatbelt injury is often followed by CT scan to assess the presence of any intra-abdominal injury (Rose, 2004). CT scans save the hospital money, reduces follow ups and avoid unnecessary radiation exposure to patients' compared to when using FAST. As a result, FAST cannot be used alone in healthcare.

Question 3

Australians are susceptible to envenomation (poisoning from animal venom) from multiple sources and treatments available in the prehospital setting

Poisoning and envenomation by terrestrial animals is one of significant health risk and economic challenge for Australians. For instance, Australian snakes are one of the most venomous animals in the world. Other animals that pose a health risk to Australians include, ants, wasps, bees, ticks and cane toads. These animals use venom for protection and predation. Ideally, the diagnostic and treatment procedures for poisoning and envenomation are expensive and traumatize many Australians. Some of the leading snake venom includes; the tiger snake, the red-bellied black snake and brown snake. Venom induces hypotension with diminished cardiac output and subsequent decrease in heart rate. Other effects of animal venom include depletion of serum fibrionogen, marked thrombocytopenia and prolonged thrombin (Hardy, Cochrane & Allavena, 2014). Pseudonaja venom contains neurotoxins leading to respiratory muscle failure and flaccid paralysis. Other symptoms such as ptyalism, hyperemic mucous membranes, recumbency or collapse, vomiting and tachypnea might also become evident. Patients are highly encouraged to apply a firm pressure bandage or immobilize joint on either site of the bite to ease the pain. The applied bandage should not be removed until the patient reaches a major hospital. Patients' are also supposed to lay down in pre-hospital settings. Some hospitals have venom detection kit which takes 20-30 minutes. Symptomatic patients should be treated with both Brown and Tiger snake antivenom in situations where the venom detection kit in unavailable (Hardy, Cochrane & Allavena, 2014). Oxygen is administered, and a large bore of intravenous catheters is inserted. Antivenom can also be given within the first four hours after the bite.

However, antivenom therapy is effective when given during the course of 24 hours. The size of the dosage is affected by the degree of envenomation.

In order to reduce the risk of anaphylactic reaction, it is advisable to pre-medicate once before administering the first dose. This can be done by administering Adrenaline 0.01 ml/kg and steroids. It is also vital to give the affected patients supportive treatments such as circulatory, ventilation and renal support (Hardy, Cochrane & Allavena, 2014).

Insect stings & bites are treated using analgesics & antihistamines. Additionally, local ice application can aid in reducing swelling and erythema. Removal of stings is also a vital process in treating bites and stings. Specifically, supplemental oxygen should be administered as the first measure in response to scorpion stings. This should be followed by administration of epinephrine in major hospitals. Severe scorpion swelling can be treated by administering one-liter fluid bolus of normal saline often followed by 5 mg of morphine sulfate intravenously (Hardy, Cochrane & Allavena, 2014).

Seemingly, marine animals such as jelly fish, sea anemones and fire corals inject toxins whenever their bite human being using stinging cells called nematocysts. Other marine animals such as sea urchins and stingrays inject their venom deeper into the tissue causing envenomation and trauma. These stings can be treated using salt waters, opioids, antihistamines and placing the affected areas in warm water. Nematocyst can also be removed using stingEze, ethanol vinegar and antivenin (Hardy, Cochrane & Allavena, 2014).

Question 4

Patients over the age of 55 who experience trauma are at risk of unrecognized major injury and, as a result, fail to receive or receive delayed care for injuries compared to younger trauma victims. Discussion of the evidence related to recognition of major injuries in elder trauma patients.

Traumatic injuries are often more severe in older adults due to lack of the right level of care. These old adults fail to seek medication in trauma centers instead opting for facilities which lack specialized expertise in treating all injuries. The leading cause of traumatic injuries among the aging population is unintentional fall. These falls are dangerous especially to those people past the age of 65 years and can lead to brain injuries and hip fractures. Patients with severe injuries should be taken to trauma center commonly found in hospital emergency departments. Additionally, motor vehicle collision and blunt injury can lead to death in elderly people. According to The Centers for Disease Control and Prevention, more than 2.3 million cases of injuries occur among old adults costing about $30 billion in direct medical care (Kristan et al., 2013). Some researchers argue that the majority of elderly patients are undertriaged and are not taken to trauma centers even though their injuries are severe enough for such attention. This can be attributed to lack awareness, resources or cultural limitations common to aging people as opposed to the young generation.

Symptoms of injury are non-specific in elderly people and are often confused with other complications emanating from their old age. For instance, altered mental status, fever, edema, increased heart rate are common in aging populations compared to young people. The occurrence of such conditions among the elderly are perceived as normal to them.

Notably, many people who fall develop a fear of falling. This reduces the mobility and the loss of physical fitness hence increasing the actual risk of falling. It is advisable for aging people to exercise regularly and focus at increasing their balance and leg strength. Additionally, Tai Chi programs are essential in improving physical fitness (Kristan et al., 2013).

Elderly people are encouraged to ask their pharmacists and doctors to review their prescription in order to reduce taking drugs with potential effects of drowsiness and dizziness. Further, their eyes should be checked at least once on an annual basis and update their eyeglasses so as to maximize their vision. According to Kristan et al. (2013), reducing tripping hazards can make homes safer and hence prevent unnecessary falls. Also, improving lighting at homes, adding railing at both sides of the stairways and adding grab bar inside and outside the tub will lower the risk of falling by a big percentage among the elderly peoples. Legislation can also help in developing strategies capable of reducing injuries. Some of this legislation includes usage of seatbelt, helmet, child car seat and alcohol control.

Kristan et al. (2013) believe that elderly people should get adequate vitamin D and calcium from supplements or diet in order to strengthen their bones. Lack of such mineral makes bone fragile and hence the risk of fall. They should also get screened for osteoporosis, which is the major of falls among the elderly people. Trauma in elderly people can be managed by using stabilization techniques, spinal immobilization, and rapid transportation of the severely injured people to hospitals. Surgery can also be deemed necessary depending on the degree of injury (Kristan et al., 2013). All these complications associated with old age reduce attention and hence poor response to their trauma compared to young people.

References

Hardy, M., Cochrane, J., & Allavena, R. (2014). Venomous and Poisonous Australian Animals of Veterinary Importance: A Rich Source of Novel Therapeutics. *BioMed Research International, 2014*, 1-12.

Kristan, L et al. (2013). Triage of Elderly Trauma Patients: A Population-Based Perspective. *Journal of the American College of Surgeons, 217*(4), 569.

Rose, J. (2004). Ultrasound in abdominal trauma. *Emerg Med Clin N Am., 22*, 581–599. Retrieved from http://www.medschool.lsuhsc.edu/emergency_medicine/docs/fast.pdf

Søreide, E & Deakin, C. (2005). Pre-hospital fluid therapy in the critically injured patient—a clinical update. *Injury, Int. J. Care Injured., 36*, 1001—1010. Retrieved from http://campus.unibo.it/70405/1/Pre-hospital_fluid_therapy_in_the_critically_injured_patient--a_clinical_update.pdf

YOUR KNOWLEDGE HAS VALUE

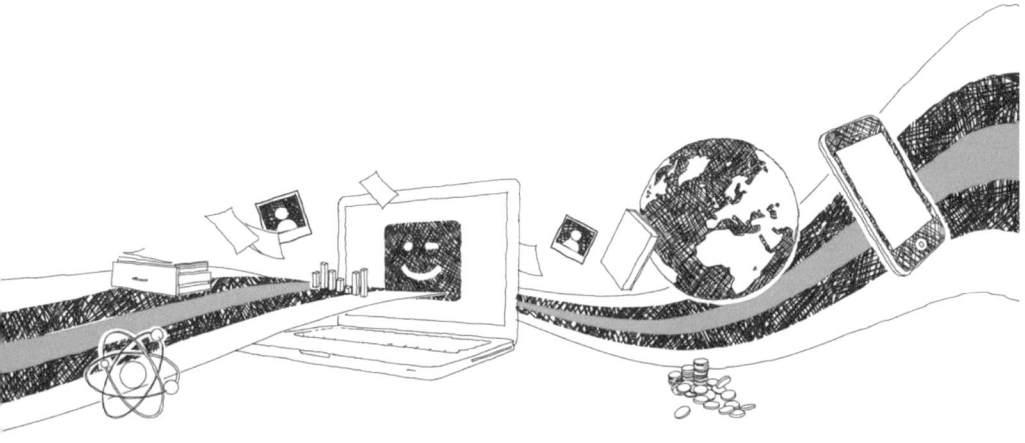

- We will publish your bachelor's and master's thesis, essays and papers

- Your own eBook and book -
  sold worldwide in all relevant shops

- Earn money with each sale

Upload your text at www.GRIN.com
and publish for free

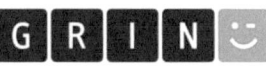